HOW TO EFT YOUR PAIN AWAY

Suzanne Zacharia

ISBN-10: 1499355033
ISBN-13: 978-1499355031

I dedicate this book to my beloved aunt, Rosette Obeid, who has asked me to write it, my children who gave me amazing support, my lovely Facebook friends who suggested titles for this book, and my spouse, who got out of the wheelchair and crutches with the help of EFT.

And to you, dear reader! You may be reading this book for yourself or as a qualified EFT/Tapping Practitioner looking for new thoughts and ideas with which to help your clients. Either way, thank you for taking the time to read and use this book.

Last but not least, I dedicate this book to all my lovely clients.

CONTENTS

HOW TO EFT YOUR PAIN AWAY

Suzanne Zacharia

CHAPTER 1 – A CURSE OR GIFT?

"Most people will do more to avoid pain than to seek pleasure" - Chris Knight. Indeed, there is a multi-million industry based on pain avoidance and management.

And there is little worse than feeling constantly or regularly in real, physical, pain.

Pain also is connected with mobility, being able to work, study, concentrate, or enjoy life properly. This could mean anything from being unable to turn your head to one side to being doubled up with IBS pain to being wheelchair-bound. Pain is connected to days off work, not being able to look after one's family, and simply having a restricted life.

We all have aches and pains from time to time. Whether you have just over-done the housework/gym/gardening or have long-term arthritis, IBS, migraine, fibromyalgia, MS, or any kind of pain, you can find something useful in this guide.

Pain is there for a reason. Acute pain is pain that has just happened recently and signals the need for immediate attention. A trip to a good Osteopath, Chiropractor, Massage Therapist, Physiotherapist, Physical Therapist, Biokineticist, Nutritionist, Kinesiologist, Allergy Specialist, Specialist Consultant Physician, Dentist, or Doctor, may be needed.

In this case, pain is there to signal the need to do something very soon. And as long as you do, there is no need for the pain to be as strong anymore. For example, if you have bad toothache, once you make an appointment to see the dentist about fixing the cause of the pain, then you have the opportunity of managing the pain until you can get to the dentist.

Chronic pain is pain that has been there for a while. Sometimes this is on-and-off over the years and sometimes it is always there. You have probably done everything that you could about it. So if it remains or returns, it may be a sign that you need a better corrective program, or it could be that the body is giving you pain signals that you can do nothing else about. In other words, in this case, the pain can be unnecessary.

If the pain is not serving a needed purpose, your body is going into overdrive, giving you all these unnecessary, or unnecessarily high, pain signals.

This may be a sign that you need to offload something which bothers your body, or to relieve your body of anything that could be overloading it.

This body overload can be physical or emotional. And of course, there is an emotional component to almost every physical symptom.

Pain management is the one tool in your life toolbox that can make life so much better. And pain management with EFT Tapping has helped more clients than I can count. Also myself, of course.

CHAPTER 2 – SHARON - YEARS OF PAIN GONE IN ONE SESSION

Way back in 2004, I was a massage therapist, Reiki practitioner, and hypnotherapist who had just qualified as an EFT practitioner. I was blown away at how EFT helped me manage my then neck pain, releasing the need for painkillers, and I wanted to share this gift with the world. One of the first clients that I shared it with was Sharon.

Sharon opened my mind to the possibilities with EFT Tapping, and her story has helped people all over the world to try EFT Tapping for their pain. By the way, I call it EFT Tapping to distinguish it from other versions that do not use tapping (a gentle form of acupressure). The main reason is that the scientific research has been carried out with the version that uses acupressure. I like dealing with something that has plenty of evidence supporting it. All my clients were offered EFT, which I refer to in this book as |EFT, EFT Tapping, or simply as tapping. Sharon was one of the first.

Sharon came into the shop where I had a clinic upstairs asking for a massage, and I just happened to have given a massage incorporating EFT to the shop owner, which he loved. He persuaded her to try my new massage. And I am so glad he did.

In the initial consultation, Sharon revealed that her life was not what it used to be. She reported a cold that just would not go away, stress headaches, eczema, sore knees, and a dull ache in the legs. She had tried massage before, and it helped somewhat.

When I asked Sharon if she had any back pain, she said yes. I checked with her the intensity of the back pain, on a scale of 10 to zero, where 10 is the most and 0 is not there. Sharon replied it was a 7 out of 10, and that it was pretty much always a 7 out of 10. I decided to offer Sharon EFT before she lay down on the massage couch, mainly because I did not want her to suffer lying down on her back, even though I always gave back support pillows.

After explaining EFT briefly, Sharon was happy to try it. I did the tapping (the EFT acupressure) on myself as she copied me, and I led her with EFT statements designed to relieve pain. She tapped on herself and repeated the statements after me as we tapped. It took only minutes for the pain to reduce to a 3 out of 0.

This in itself is a great result. I could have stopped there but felt that there was more to this pain. I asked Sharon how long she had had this particular pain. She replied

hat she had it for four years. And that her life had gone downhill ever since the pain had started. I asked what had happened in her life just before the onset of this back pain.

She then told me that this was since she had a car accident. She was stopped at a traffic light when the other driver slammed into the back of her car. A lightbulb suddenly turned on in my mind. There it was!

SO, I suggested that this trauma had somehow kept the pain going and asked for permission to release this trauma. Sharon agreed. We proceeded to tap (do EFT) for the trauma. The pain almost completely disappeared. So I asked Sharon, if there was an emotion still stuck in her back, what would it be? She replied that it was anger at the other driver. We tapped for this anger, with the **emphasis being that it was not to relieve the other driver of the blame, but for Sharon's pain to go.** And the pain reduced to zero.

I then proceeded on to the massage. Since Sharon had received massages before, and they had only helped a little for a short period of time, I believe that it was the EFT Tapping that made the difference.

Sharon saw me again for about 5 sessions. She reported starting work again, going back to the gym, and no more of the pesky physical symptoms that she used to have. The back pain did not return, not even a year later.

Many thanks to Sharon, who was happy to share her experience with you and spread the word.

EFT is a very versatile tool literally at your fingertips. We stimulate easy-to-reach acupressure points (by tapping on them with our fingers) whilst repeating specially-targeted phrases. Although this case was mainly about back pain, the EFT Tapping process is the same for pretty much any type of pain, from migraines to IBS. EFT is like a pill you can take whenever you want, without side effects. It literally is pain management at your fingertips.

Sharon got rid of all her pain in minutes, and it did not come back. Will it happen for you too? I do not know, but I do know that EFT has helped me and many, many clients for over two decades.

CHAPTER 3 –
"ABRAHAM" – A
CONSTANT HEADACHE
FOR A YEAR GONE
IN ONE SESSION

When I first learned EFT, I used it for my then neck pain. I tapped (did EFT) every 3-4 hours, bringing the pain from a 9 out of 10 to a zero every time. I did it for 3 months before one day, I woke up without this pain. I still needed to tap for the pain maybe a few times a week after that, and some weeks or months later, I realized that I had not noticed the pain for some time. On the other hand, "Abraham" (not his real name), like Sharon, completely got rid of his pain in one session. I, and he, were overjoyed!

Abraham had initially seen me for a massage as a gift from his wife. During the initial consultation, it transpired that he had a constant headache since a year before. Abraham could not think of anything physical or emotional that had happened to him before the headache started. He also assured me that the matter was thoroughly medically investigated, and that he was seeing his medical professionals regularly to ensure there was nothing sinister to be addressed. Since the massage was a gift, I then gave him the requested massage without any EFT. However, I also mentioned that I had a forthcoming EFT Tapping workshop for pain management and invited him to attend.

Abraham enrolled in the workshop. It was a small class, so we were able to spend a few hours in a leisurely way. He first learned about the background of EFT Tapping. Then the tapping points were introduced and the statements explained in full. This was followed by a practice run, where we did not direct EFT onto the pain but just practiced doing the tapping points whilst saying practice statements. As a side-note, I find that doing a practice run is very useful for someone who has never enjoyed a meridian therapy before, such as a good acupuncture or Shiatsu treatment. Experience has taught me that it is worth spending quality time learning about EFT tapping and doing a practice run before using it on a real issue. This is why this book contains the foundational practice run and explanations of EFT and about pain. Put it this way, I would not do anything if you simply tell me to, and I would not expect you to either! I need evidence and background, so that I can make an informed decision.

When the time came to learn EFT Tapping for pain, we measured the intensity of pain that the attendees were experiencing at that moment in time. Then we started tapping, re-assessing the level of pain on a scale of 10 to 0 after each round (iteration) of EFT. Abraham's numbers went down and continued going down till they were soon at a 0 level of pain.

At different later times in the workshop, I checked with Abraham to see what his headache pain level was. It remained at a zero. And it remained at a zero even a month later when I followed up.

Whilst it is not the norm in my experience that headaches and migraines disappear in one session, I hope that Abraham's story gives you the motivation to try EFT for your pain.

And remember that although this case was mainly about a persistent headache, the EFT Tapping process is the same for pretty much any type of pain. What I love about EFT is its simplicity. Pain management does not have to be complicated.

CHAPTER 4 –
RESEARCH EVIDENCE

This is one of various studies conducted by top EFT researchers. They found that "EFT may modulate stress to reduce chronic pain."

Two groups of of a total of 147 people with physical pain participated in the study. Two groups received a 2-hour EFT Tapping session weekly for six weeks. In one group, two qualified EFT practitioners conducted the sessions via Zoom calls. In the second group, people did the same but using pre-recorded sessions. And the third group acted as a control group; they were put on a waiting list and did not receive EFT during these six weeks.

The results are for the people who completed the 6-week program.

Measures for pain severity and interference of pain with activities were equally significantly lower than the pretreatment scores for the two groups who had received the EFT. The control group (who did not receive EFT during these six weeks) did not show a difference.

To quote: "These findings offer early promise for EFT as a potentially effective pain management strategy" and "growing body of literature presenting EFT as a potentially effective pain management strategy with very little downside."

If you wish to see the full paper, this is the reference:
Stapleton, P., Wilson, C., Uechtritz, N., Stewart, M., McCosker, M.,

O'Keefe, T., & Blanchard, M. (2025). A randomized clinical trial of emotional freedom techniques for chronic pain: Live versus self-paced delivery with 6-month follow-up. European Journal of Pain, 29(3), e4740.

CHAPTER 5 - DEFINITION AND TYPES OF PAIN

We have already discussed acute versus chronic pain, whereby acute pain is pain that happened fairly recently and chronic is pain that started some time ago, and in some cases, many years. EFT Tapping does not make anyone silly. Nor does it take away the protective action of pain. For example, if someone has just had a successful operation on their knee, and they experience an expected post-operative pain (acute pain), the EFT Tapping can help reduce or even release the pain. However, if this person tries to kneel on that knee the day after the operation, they will feel pain and (if they are sensible enough) choose not to kneel at such an early stage after the operation. If someone experiences back pain regularly for years (chronic pain), the EFT Tapping can help reduce, manage, or even release the pain. Those are my observations from over 20 years of experience with clients.

We also have 2 more types of pain.

Nociceptive pain is an ordinary response to tissue damage, such as an injury or a burn. For example, if you sprain your ankle. Nociceptive pain is typically a response to something detected by certain pain receptors called nociceptors in the affected area. When the nociceptors are activated, they send signals via the spinal cord up to the brain, which interprets these signals as pain.

This pain can have qualities of being sharp, aching, or throbbing, and it is typically in a particular area, such as the ankle, in the case of a sprained ankle. It may occur with injury or inflammation.

Now, EFT Tapping has been linked to something in our cells that is connected to "regulation of 6 genes associated with inflammation ". If you would like to know more, the source is Maharaj ME. Differential gene expression after Emotional Freedom Techniques (EFT) treatment: a novel pilot protocol for salivary mRNA assessment. Energy Psychol Theory Res Treat. 2016;8(1):17–32. doi:10.9769/EPJ.2016.8.1.MM

In my experience with physical pain clients, it helps to be specific when using EFT Tapping, by expressing what the pain feels like and where it is. And since much pain involves inflammation, it helps to be specific with inflammation, too.

For example, instead of simply saying "this pain" when you tap to relieve or release it, you can say "this pain in my ankle", "this throbbing pain in my ankle", "this sharp pain in my ankle", or "this inflammation in my ankle".

If you are new to EFT Tapping, just come back to this chapter after you learn how to tap more simply for pain, and you will then see how to apply statements such as those above, in order to be more specific.

Inflammation can also be part of a nerve pain. Neuropathic pain is the type of pain to do with the actual nerves. It is a symptom of a malfunction of, or injury to, certain nerves of the nervous system. The causes include injury, disease, or a condition that affects the nervous system, such as diabetes, multiple sclerosis, or an accident. The damage done to the nerves can lead to abnormal pain signaling. Nerve damage can cause pain to be felt even when we have not sprained our ankle, for example. And the nerves can become overly sensitive, leading to pain for no apparent resaon.

This type of pain can have qualities of burning, tingling, shooting, stabbing, a numbness, or a weakness in a particular area.

As above, in my experience with physical pain clients, it helps to be specific when using EFT Tapping, by saying what the pain feels like, and where it is. And since much pain involves inflammation, it helps to be specific with inflammation, too.

For example, instead of simply saying "this pain" when you tap to manage it, you can say "this pain in my left leg", "this shooting pain in my left leg", "this stabbing pain in my left leg", "this numbness in my arm", "this weakness in my legs", or "this inflamed nerve in my leg".

This chapter was especially written in layman's language and style, in order to be easy to read. However, it still is more of a nice-to-have rather than a need-to-master. If you are new to EFT Tapping, just come back to this chapter after you learn how to tap more simply for pain, and you will then have a clear idea of how to apply more specific statements such as those above.

CHAPTER 6 - HOW OUR NERVOUS SYSTEM PROCESSES PAIN SIGNALS

Let us look at how sensory receptors, neural pathways, and the brain together process the pain signals. You may ask if this is needed for you to release or relieve your own pain, and no, it is not; but if you are curious, or if you are a practitioner wanting to know more, I feel that this is useful to learn.

The nociceptors are all over, such as in our skin, muscles, joints, organs, and the brain. When something activates a nociceptor, it triggers an electrical signal that travels along the nerve fibers to the spinal cord. Here, the pain signals can either be transmitted directly to the brain, or it can be first processed at a local level for a necessary immediate reflex action (for example, moving your hand away if you have accidentally touched a hot stove).

Pain signals travel through a pathway that goes up via the spinal cord toward the brainstem and then to the thalamus, the brain's relay center for sensory information. The pain signals may be modified, for example, by inhibitory pathways that can reduce our perception of pain (this seems to be what happens when you rub something to make it feel better).

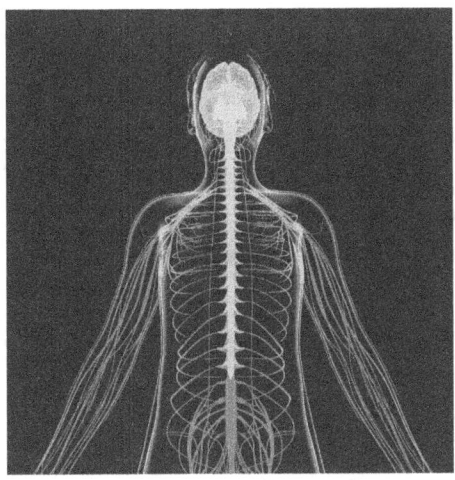

Once the pain signals reach the thalamus, they go to other areas of the brain for interpretation. One such area is the somatosensory cortex, which tells us where the pain is, such as in the right ankle.

Another such brain area is the limbic system. This is involved in emotions and memory. So it makes sense that pain is not just a physical feeling but also an emotional feeling. For example, pain can make us feel short-tempered, fearful, or anxious. Also, these emotional responses can make the physical pain seem worse. The pain can feel like it is shouting if we are very stressed, whereas otherwise, it would only be a whisper.

Another brain area, the prefrontal cortex, helps us to assess whether the pain is dangerous or just a temporary nuisance, so we can respond appropriately. For example, if we feel too much heat coming from a hot stove, we make the decision not to touch it, and if we simply feel a little bit hot on a summer's day, we may just put up with it.

Pain modulation is the body regulating or adjusting the intensity and perception of physical pain. The brain can either amplify or dampen pain signals depending on factors such as our emotions and previous experiences. For example, feeling really stressed can make pain feel worse. And EFT Tapping is a great way to de-stress.

Pain is modulated via pathways going down from the brain to the spinal cord. These pathways release **neurotransmitters such as serotonin and endorphins, which, in effect, inhibit the transmission of pain signals.** And there is also the **gate control theory, which suggests that a light touch or pressure can "close the gate" to pain signals, preventing them from reaching the brain.** This is why rubbing a sore spot can sometimes provide relief. I do wonder if it also why tapping works for pain.

CHAPTER 7 –
CHRONIC PAIN AND
NEUROPLASTICITY

With chronic pain, the nervous system may become way too sensitive. Pain signals can be amplified or misinterpreted, for example with fibromyalgia, neuropathic pain, and chronic back pain for which people take way too many painkillers. With chronic pain, the pain pathways can become overactive.

Neuroplasticity is the brain's ability to reorganize and form new neural connections,. The brain can "rewire" itself in response to persistent pain, making the sensation of pain more constant. The central nervous system can get caught up in this heightened pain sensitivity, creating a vicious cycle.

We can also create good neuroplastic changes, leading to pain relief. Pain can be unlearned, released, or relieved through neuroplasticity. The brain can be retrained to reduce pain sensitivity.

CHAPTER 8 – YOUR OPTIMAL WELL-BEING

Optimal well-being means living your best life that you can under the given circumstances. EFT Tapping may completely get rid of your pain, or it can be a wonderful method of pain management that you can use for free, without nasty side-effects, at any time you want.

This book is a simple guide based on new and far-reaching concepts. It does not take the place of medical advice and is not intended as advice. This is simply how to use EFT Tapping for pain management according to my extensive skills and experience in the field.

And now for some disclaimers...

Kindly assume responsibility for your own physical and mental wellbeing. People with schizophrenia or psychosis are not usually suited for EFT. If in doubt, ask your medical professional. Remember, this is for your optimal well-being.

This book assumes that you have already gotten medical attention and there is nothing else the medical system can do for your pain.

Regardless of the above proviso, you are advised to consult with your physician before embarking on any alternative, complementary, beauty, or self-help regime.

Our use of systems that are trademarked or have a registered trademark represents our views and not necessarily those of the trademark owners.

Please be aware that this book cannot be taken as massage practitioner, physiotherapist, oncologist, chiropractor, nutritionist, herbalist, or any other such professional's advice. Nor is it a substitute for supervision for Practitioners, unless your association clearly states that it can be used as such, or as CPD.

This book is not designed as, nor is it a replacement for, medical advice.

And now onto some things that your medical practitioner may not know about your pain. The following chapter lays out some sub-clinical factors from my client experience.

CHAPTER 9 - WHAT IS ALSO BOTHERING YOUR BODY?

Your bones, muscles, organs, and the nerves that carry signals to and from your painful body parts are all made up from what you eat, drink, and otherwise assimilate into your body. If your body hurts, it may be that what you have, or have not, eaten or drunk has something to do with it.

There are substances and situations that are often found to be culprits. The following is a small collection of some common suspected baddies.

Wheat/gluten. Gluten is the stuff that holds bread together, a bit like glue or wallpaper paste. And maybe it is not such a good idea to eat lots of gluey stuff daily if it bothers your body.

Artificial sweeteners are suspected by some of being a nerve toxin and so may increase pain.

Anything which acts as a stimulant to the nervous system can increase pain.

Bloatedness can be uncomfortable and clog your system. We can get bloated if we develop a reaction to a food substance. As well as finding out what it is, variety is good. If your body is likely to develop a reaction to something, it is more likely to develop a reaction to something it is over-exposed to. Eating the same food almost daily is not a good idea unless you are on a safe elimination diet given by a qualified nutritionist, for example.

Too much sugar (including anything starchy or sweet), beer, or wine, invites organisms that kind of attack your body and reduce your immunity. One of the most common culprits is Candida albicans, which you may or may not have heard of. I have found this to be a factor in clients with many conditions, including Rheumatoid Arthritis. The modern diet has too much sugar in any case, and drinking too much is a big problem in many countries.

Could you have Lyme Disease? This may he hard to detect and some doctors do have an effective, if extreme, treatment. Do an internet search everything you can if this is a suspicion. You can also see a good functional medicine naturopath/doctor, bioresonance, or kinesiology practitioner.

Are you overweight or underweight? This can affect the musculo-skeletal system, your lymph, your circulation, and just about every bodily organ. For example, eating too little can affect a woman's hormone levels and lead to osteoporosis. And eating too much adds more weight for your body to carry and less circulation around squeezed organs inside your body.

Could your body be suffering from a bad posture or lack of appropriate movement?

Do you grind your teeth at night, causing jaw, neck, and shoulder pain?

EFT Tapping can help with an element of all the above. For example, if you have a multigrain breakfast with toast for breakfast, a sandwich for lunch, and pasta for dinner, and it has been found that you have a sub-clinical problem with wheat, you can tap to release the need to have it at more than one meal a day (or as otherwise recommended by your practitioner).

What I really would love to do is to show you now, right now, how you can be free of this pain forever, but experience has shown me that it is best to explain the background thoroughly first, let it sink in, and then the pain sufferer can much more easily let go of that pain. I myself knew about EFT for a year whilst I suffered the most excruciating pain and needed a year's convincing before I finally tried it.

There are whole industries built around pain. Everything from painkillers to creams and lotions to machines to massages... The list is endless, and every now and then, there is a new patch or magnetic device or some other gizmo designed for pain relief. But could it be that you are also suffering from an emotional compnent? Physical pain is very real. If you put your hand on the muscles involved, you can feel the tension. Shooting pains, such as with sciatica for example, can be felt all night, keeping the sufferer awake tossing and turning. A frozen shoulder can only move so far and anyone can literally see the range of movement is limited. How can that not be physical?! That is not all in the head. However, I found a method of pain release that has the power of releasing even the pain of a permanent back injury. This method is our friend EFT, short for Emotional Freedom Techniques.

As you may know, my first encounter with EFT Tapping for back and excruciating neck pain (and the ensuing headaches) was my own, which was initially released in minutes. It came back every 3-4 hours, and I simply tapped it away in minutes. It was much faster than taking an anti-inflammatory or pain-killer tablet and reduced the pain down to a zero rather than a 4 out of ten. I still believed it was a physical thing and refused to consider that there was an emotional component. However, **after finally addressing all the underlying emotional issues from the past that were somehow stuck in that area**, I am now permanently pain-free despite a permanent real physical challenge in my upper back. A small version of the pain comes back maybe once or twice a year when I am extremely **stressed** or on the rare occasion when I physically injure myself in that area again, but the pain does not last long, because I tap it away and take all necessary steps to get rid of all its physical components, including boring rehabilitation exercises. And boring rehabilitation exercises become very interesting with the help of EFT!

And you have read about the case of Sharon, who released back pain of four years' duration in one session once the emotional component was collapsed. The back pain was somehow due to holding onto anger for the driver who had caused the accident leading to the pain in the first place. Once this anger was released, the pain was completely gone - permanently. After this experience, I became a believer that our emotions can be a significant component of back pain.

So even when there is an actual permanent physical component to the pain, it is the emotional component that keeps the chronic pain there. Sometimes, the physical weakness in that area makes it susceptible to being like a holding vessel for any fresh negative emotions that would otherwise trouble us. In other words, the emotions stuck in that painful part of your body, be it your head, knee, back, foot, tummy, or wherever. And I identify an emotion as any reaction of your mind-body to anything that bothers it, including toxins in your environment, anger, fear, resentment, guilt, shame, foods that cause your body inflammation, and so on. The release of this emotional component is now made possible with EFT Tapping.

The next chapter clarifies how EFT Tapping can be different to other pain approaches. A different way of thinking can open up a whole new path to comfort and peace.

CHAPTER 10 - A DIFFERENT APPROACH WITH EFT TAPPING

We all want to be strong and healthy. And what feeling can be nicer than triumph in the face of adversity? To fight and win is exhilarating!

Whether physically or emotionally, strength is highly desirable. Sometimes strength comes naturally from within, and sometimes we have to work at it. And one instance where we need to be strong, for example, is when we have a physical mishap. Take shoulder pain, for example. The average person that wakes up with a little pain in the shoulder will try to ignore it. And it usually goes away.

It is common to ignore a little pain in the shoulders, after all.

Many feel that if we ignore it, this is a sign of strength. But in my experience, an ignored ache or discomfort can lead to some or all of the following.

The body compensates for the discomfort by putting undue stress in previously healthy muscles and joints, thereby causing the problem to spread elsewhere in the body.

People often take painkillers when the pain becomes a real nuisance. But painkillers have side effects, and

continued use of painkillers has been implicated
in stomach problems, for example.

Pain also leads to increased irritability. This in turn leads to
reduced performance in one's work, leisure, and personal life.

Pain can reduce the quality of sleep. Even what begins as a
discomfort can suddenly become a pain just before bedtime.

So maybe admitting to an ache or discomfort is acceptable, when
you do so in order to address the pain. Tight muscles, overused
joints, stress on the mind and body, carrying something heavy,
even shopping, can take its toll on our bodies. We all get aches and
discomforts. Sometimes it is good to take time for ourselves and
relax.

In the experience of most people, negative feelings and sensations
need to be ignored, and as we think positively, we can be positive
in the face of any adversity. Ignoring the pain and forcing yourself
to do a full day at work, ignoring the pain and carrying on with a
grueling sport, this is often seen as a sign of strength.

Hidden negative emotions are found to be surfacing as a
contributing cause of physical manifestations, such as back ache,
migraines, or IBS. For most people, this is a sign that we need to
ignore these feelings even more.

But if we ignore negative emotions that have somehow overtaken
our bodies and increased physical pain unnecessarily, does not
mean that we have removed them! It only means that we have a
coping strategy.

A coping strategy is a good thing. Sometimes, although we can be
truly find respite or even freedom from pain, this may take time,
in which case a good coping strategy is wise in the meantime.
For an increasing number of truly blessed individuals, there is
the discovery that pain can be managed or released. And when
the pain is gotten under control, the mind-body naturally feels
relaxation and contentment.

Remember; it takes a great deal of strength to allow relaxation. But relaxation makes you stronger! To achieve this relaxation effectively, you need a quick and simple method that you can easily use whenever needed. EFT Tapping is just such a tool.

EFT Tapping is somehow used for physical pain, emotional feelings, substances, and germs that can disrupt your energy system. In the case of some germs, I personally think that the medical route is better. However, when all medical routes are exhausted, that is when people come to me for Tapping sessions as a last resort. And we often achieve amazing results. I use the Allergy Antidotes system for substances and germs. If you would like to look it up and get more knowledge, this is the Allergy Antidotes website: www.allergyantidotes.com.

A good thing to work on is the "emotional" part of the issue. And here I define an emotion as your body's reaction to anything that bothers it.

As well as substances that can bother your body, emotions around safety can appear. You may well ask, is it safe to get rid of your pain? EFT feels like a great idea, but you may well ask about the wisdom of losing pain. For example, what if the pain is due to something that needs urgent attention? Is it safe to do EFT for pain due to a potential fracture requiring urgent medical attention? Well, one great bonus of using EFT for pain is its safety. Let me illustrate with an example.

I was treating clients in a workshop for their back pain. One in particular did not respond to the tapping at all. Her pain was still something like an 8 out of 10. So I sat next to her and asked her more questions about her pain. From her answers, I gathered that her pain was acute and needed urgent manipulation to prevent further injury. Still trying to be helpful, I gave her the number of a top chiropractor that I knew would take good care of her and made her promise to make an appointment with him the next day. And then I thought to tap anyway, to conclude our work. We tapped whilst saying something like:

"Even though I have this pain, I promise to make the appointment with the osteopath tomorrow. I deeply love and accept myself".

To my astonishment, this lady's pain started to fade away! So we continued tapping like that, and in minutes the pain went down to a more manageable 3 out of 10. It would not go down further. This implied to me that necessary pain does not begin to fade with EFT Tapping unless we make a plan to address its causes.

And I have come across numerous occasions since where a pain that was needed did not go away with EFT. So EFT is not a method of superficial pain relief or pain management but a holistic pain solution.

"Truly thank you, Suzanne, for helping me achieve freedom from more than 25 years of pain with EFT in your class. 14 months after your class, I'm still free from my pain" - Sejual

CHAPTER 11 - EASY PRACTICE ROUND

If you are totally familiar with EFT Tapping, you can easily just skip this chapter. Otherwise, read on.

What is EFT?

EFT is an "Energy Healing", "Meridian Tapping Technique (MTT)", or "Tapping" method. It is used by many as a self-help method for any emotional or physical condition. Used by practitioners of many different modalities, from physiotherapy and personal training to medicine to hypnotherapy, to enhance their therapy toolkit, it is also used as a standalone practice by a growing number of specialist EFT practitioners worldwide. You may be new to EFT, or it may be a familiar friend already. Either way, you can learn EFT very easily from the most loved version in this book.

EFT works on the principle that what causes undesirable feelings is a disruption in the body's energy system. This disruption includes various elements of our biochemistry and nervous system. For simplicity, I will refer to it all as "energy", because that is the all-encompassing term used in the complementary therapy and self-help world.

This energy is the same energy that various therapies talk about, including acupuncture, Reiki, and Shiatsu.

In essence, when we do EFT, we:

Remove the "wrong" energy from our body by using the

meridian lines as a kind of waste disposal system.

Access this "wrong" energy to be removed by calling it up.

So, when we do EFT, we:

Tap on important points in the body's meridian system.

Call up the waste energy to be disposed of by saying a
Reminder phrase. This is after setting up the process
safely and gently using a Setup phrase.

This is like:

Your waste disposal people come to collect your household waste.

In order for them to do so, you pick it up and
put it out for them to collect.

It is important to understand that in EFT we only **briefly** connect
to the negative. We safely and gently dispose of it. And to dispose
of it, we need to safely collect it and throw it away.

This is so effective that sometimes, people forget they ever had a
problem with something in the first place.

This book uses my own specialist adaptations of EFT, with
illustrations to help you as you go along. To see The EFT tapping
points used in motion (and my many nuances thereof), just go
to my easy instructional YouTube free EFT Tapping course on my
website. There are videos of me doing EFT here, and you can view
them as often as you wish free of charge:
https://youtube.com/playlist?
list=PLgXEZyXpeQERk_EL_OKDug6LyrhNPk9PF&si=2TFkVisuFP
_x6ILs

To see the link, you may have to type it into your browser,
depending on whether you have bought the paperback or Kindle,
for example.

Easier still, you can visit my YouTube channel here: https://www.youtube.com/@EFT-Tapping-Course-and-Videos – all new visitors are directed to the first part of the EFT Tapping course. The link to each next class is always in the Description section under the video. Very easy!

Most importantly, you can try EFT yourself as soon as the opportunity arises. Do not only read this book. Do this book. Get rid of that pain, manage that pain, get in control of that pain, as much as you can. Use this great skill at your fingertips to make life easier. Give it a good try and see what you think.

OK, now let's do a practice EFT Tapping round (iteration).

I will explain to you all the points you need to use. Then we will do a dummy run. Then we will start the EFT process.

We start each round of tapping with a Setup phrase said 3 times, unless otherwise specified. We continue the round saying a Reminder phrase. Experienced EFTers may prefer to do the Setup only once to save time, as it is often not needed 3 times. However, most tappers enjoy doing it 3 times and find comfort in this.

You can use one hand or the other for tapping, or even both, if you prefer. We tap with at least two fingers and preferably all. If you have nice long nails, just tap with the pads of your fingers to avoid bruising yourself with your nails.

The EFT acupressure points we are going to use are explained below, and then illustrated for clarity.

For the Setup phrase:
The Karate Chop (the hitting edge of your hand if playing Karate)

For the Reminder phrase:
Top of the Head (where you have a swirly thing at the crown)
Eye Brow (where the eyebrow usually meets the top of the nose)
Side of the Eye (where your eyebrow ends)
Under the Eye (on your cheekbone)

Under the Nose (between your nose and mouth)

Chin (in the middle of the horizontal line on your chin)

The mis-named Collarbone (on the bony protrusion just either side of the "V" at the bottom of your neck)

Under the Arm (under your arm where if you were female and wearing a bra, it would be the middle of the bra band)

The Setup sets up the one round of tapping. The Reminder phrase is so that you can continue kind of focused on the issue you wish freedom from. A round of EFT is a sequence of EFT going around the body once.

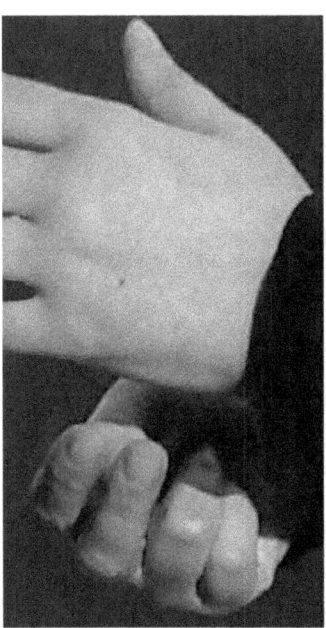

Karate Chop (the chopping edge of your hand as if playing Karate)

We tap on each point with at least two fingers. This way, we do not have to find the exact spot but cover a good area that includes the exact acupressure point.

We tap on all the points while we are saying our statements, as if tapping in time to music.

If you have a disability that precludes you from reaching or tapping on some of the points or tapping with two fingers, do not worry about it!

EFT is a very robust system. You can leave some points out and it still works. If one of these points is the Karate Chop, you can use any other point for the Setup.

And you do not need to do the points in the order presented. You can do them in whatever order you wish.

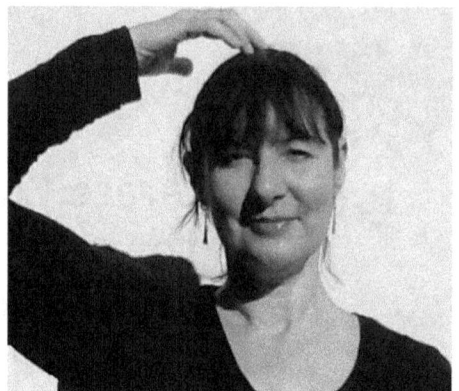

Top of the Head
(at the crown)

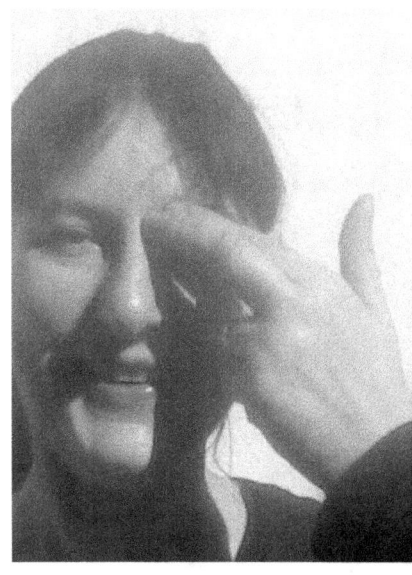

Eye Brow (where eyebrow meets top of nose)

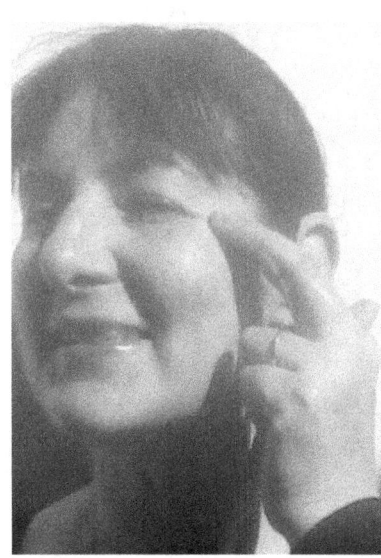

Side of Eye (just a bit further from the outside of the eye)

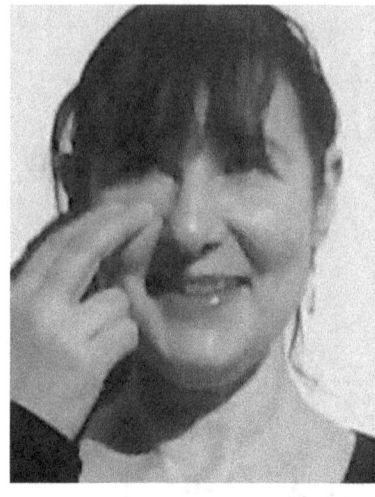

Under Eye (Straight under the eye on your cheekbone)

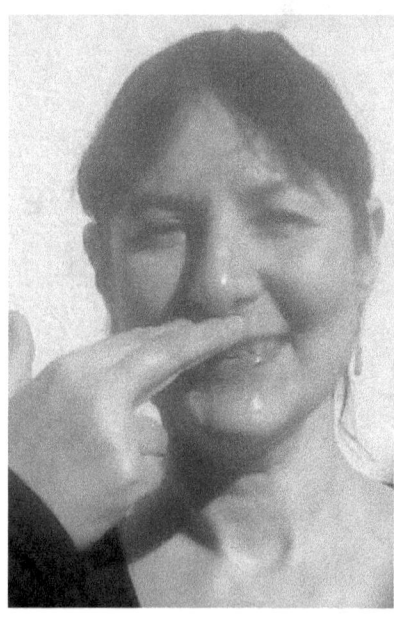

Nose (under the nose, between your nose and upper lip)

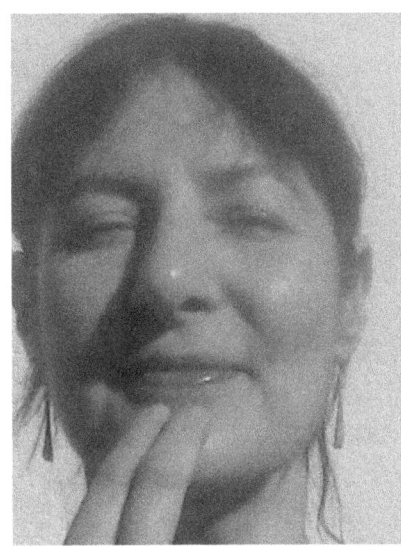

Chin (in the middle of the horizontal line on your chin)

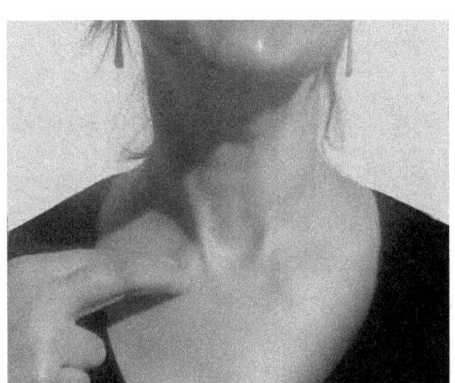

Collarbone (the end of a collarbone at the bottom of the neck)

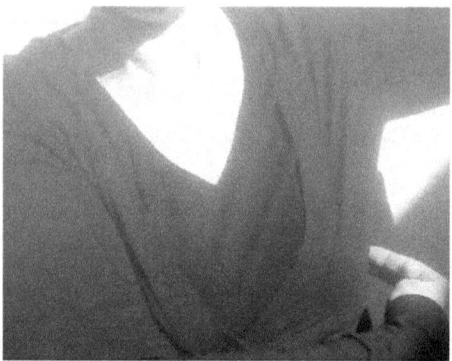

Under Arm (where the bra band would be on the side of the body)

Now let us do a "practice run" so that you will be familiar with the tapping procedure.

And Remember...

It may feel strange at first and **all** new things seem strange at first.

The reason why EFT/Tapping is taking the world by storm is just that it is such an effective self-help tool. I cannot tell with 100% certainty that it will work with you, but since it has helped so many of my clients, chances are that you will soon be seeing results too.

"Do not fear to be eccentric in opinion, for every opinion now accepted was once eccentric" - Bertrand Russell.

When/if you are already familiar with the points, just follow the tapping instructions.

You do not have to say the statements out loud. For example, if you have someone in the next room that can hear you, you may or may not wish to make them part of the experience.

You can say the statements in your head, imagining saying them out loud.

It's easy!

Tap on the Karate Chop continuously as you say this Setup statement three times.

Setup:
"Even though I'm doing this strange tapping thing, I accept myself, and that's OK, even if I don't"

Now tap on the Top of the Head continuously as you say this Reminder statement once.

Reminder:
"This strange tapping thing"

Now tap on the Eye Brow continuously as you say this Reminder statement once.

Reminder:
"This strange tapping thing"

Next tap on the Side of Eye continuously as you say this Reminder statement once.

Reminder:
"This strange tapping thing"

Now tap on the Under Eye continuously as you say this Reminder statement once.

Reminder:
"This strange tapping thing"

Next tap on the Nose point continuously as you say this Reminder statement once.

Reminder:
"This strange tapping thing"

Tap on the Chin continuously as you say this Reminder statement once.

Reminder:

"This strange tapping thing"

And now tap on the Collarbone continuously as you say this Reminder statement once.

Reminder:

"This strange tapping thing"

Next tap on the Under Arm continuously as you say this Reminder statement once.

Reminder:

"This strange tapping thing"

And that's it.

You now know how to tap on the tapping points and how to combine the acupressure with the spoken word. Well done!

CHAPTER 12 - SUDS OR LEVEL OF NEGATIVE FEELINGS

SUDS is a term for the Subjective Unit of Distress Scale, or how bad we could feel. We will be measuring the level of physical pain, craving, stress, or any negative emotions in various situations. You do not need to identify what the feeling exactly is, just get an idea of how intense it is. This is so that you can tell when it is gone down and move onto the next step.

It is very important that when we tap for physical pain, this pain is felt in the actual present moment when we tap.

Some may call their pain a discomfort. Don't let semantics get in the way of your feeling better. You call the sensation whatever you see fit. You are in control of this process.

If you are not **currently in any physical pain or discomfort**, you can learn how to tap for pain by maybe trying to touch your toes, raise your arms high, or breathe fully, in a way that is safe for you to do. Any discomfort or lack of ease (such as not having a full breath) can be used to learn how to ease a physical symptom.

If you wish to release or relieve past or future emotional situations that are somehow connected to the physical pain, then imagine how intense you would feel **if** you were to think about these situations. If these are in the present moment, simply have a guess at the intensity of negative feeling you experience.

Remember that physical pain has to be felt in the moment. If you feel no pain appearing right now, because the pain flares up, say, after eating, once a week, or on a menstrual period, you can practice by touching your toes, raising your arms high, or seeing how much you can breathe in. Then when you get an actual pain that you need to manage, you can come back to this chapter and be familiar with what to do.

Each situation you tap for has to be **specific**.

The more specific you can be, the better EFT works. For example, "This burning pain behind my right shoulder blade", "This spasming in my lower back, just there", "This feeling as if a migraine is about to come on", "This period pain", "this shooting pain in my right leg", "When visiting my friend Amy", "This inflamed nerve squeezed by my hip muscles", or "The day my colleague shouted at me".

We measure the SUDS from 10 to 0, 10 being the worst, 0 being neutral or kind of calm. We aim to get all SUDS to 0 for complete success.

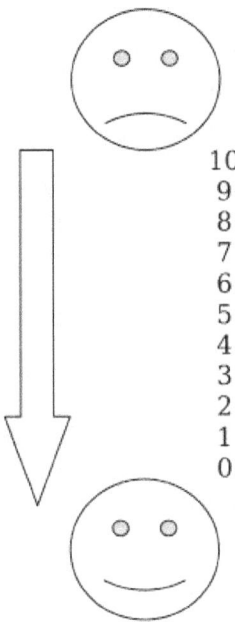

SUDS sometimes present a challenge. If this is the case, that is OK. Just rate the intensity of as feeling Small, Medium, or Large. Or you can rate it Present or Absent. Simple.

If after tapping several rounds of EFT, there is no intensity, that is OK too. It probably means zero. Figuring out your pain levels is not an exact science.

Remember, this book is not about doing EFT exactly right, it is simply about feeling better. As long as you feel better, that's all that matters.

There is no need to get yourself all worked up about "doing it right". EFT is very robust.

If you have to miss some of the acupressure points, for instance because you may have eczema on one side of your face, that's OK.

And if you keep tapping for say, 20 minutes, and the pain only goes down from a 7 out of 10 to a 5 out of 10, that is also good. If you get tired tapping or the numbers get stuck, say, at the 5 in this example, take a break. You can carry on later.

Remember that I tapped several times a day for my then pain for 3 months before the results held for longer than a day. And it was some weeks later when I noticed that I no longer needed to tap for the pain.

Each time I tapped for that pain only took about 15 minutes, faster than taking some pain relief tablets.

I was already used to taking pain relief tablets every 4 hours and waiting about 15-20 minutes for the tablets to work. It did not seem very different to tap instead.

The lack of side-effects from the medication was a wonderful unexpected gift!

Talking about the unexpected, pain management can be weird sometimes. You may find yourself experiencing a release when you tap for physical pain. This release can be via tears, laughter, giggles, or it can be via physical symptoms such as burping, or coughing. If so, just let it happen. A release could be sighing, tears, seemingly inappropriate giggles or laughter, burping, sneezing, coughing, or shaking, just to give a few examples. Keep tapping silently on any point that feels right. It is perfectly OK to feel emotion. Allow these negative emotions to surface, release, and leave your energy system.

Make sure you have a glass of water nearby, and keep filling it up. You need to drink water. EFT is thirsty work. You may find yourself breaking for the toilet, as the water has to go somewhere! That is perfectly normal.

Occasionally, a headache is experienced. That is normal. It signifies the uncomfortable "energy" is kind of trying to leave your body through your head. You can tap for the headache too. Sometimes it is a sign that you need to drink some water, as energy work like EFT can leave you feeling thirsty. You can also get up and have a stretch, and make sure you are in a comfortable, well-ventilated room.

CHAPTER 13 - LET'S TAP FOR IT

This tapping assumes that you currently have a pain or discomfort somewhere in your body. If not, you can move around a bit until you feel it. Of course, you must make sure that you do not cause yourself an injury by doing so! Or you can try the following suggestions for practice.

If you are not currently in any physical pain or discomfort, you can learn how to tap for pain by maybe trying to touch your toes, raise your arms high, or breathe fully, in a way that is safe for you to do. Any discomfort or lack of ease (such as not having a full breath) can be used to learn how to ease a physical symptom.

When you are ready, get a pen and paper, or whatever works for you to write your EFT Setup and Reminder phrases. And once you have tapped a few times, you will easily flow with the tapping and will no longer need to write anything down.

Most of us have an ache or pain somewhere. Maybe a sore back, a pain in the neck, tight shoulders, or an itch somewhere.

Of course, since this is a physical issue, how well it will respond to EFT is unknown. However, even if you could reduce a throbbing pain to a dull ache, that is a great improvement.

So, what is your pain or discomfort?

With physical issues, just like the emotional ones, we try to be as specific as possible. Some of the most frequent answers I get are:

A dull ache at the top of the right shoulder.
A pain on the outside of the left knee when getting up.
An itch on inside of the right wrist.
A stretch felt on the back of the knees when touching the toes.
A headache.
Lower back pain.
Period pain.
IBS pain.
Neck or shoulder tightness.

Let us take the discomfort of Jan, who felt an itch on the inside of the right wrist. Jan taps for "itch on the inside of my right wrist".

So, what is your physical challenge right now as you read this? Where is it exactly? Write it here:

My pain/discomfort/challenge that I feel at this very moment in time is "_____"

Take SUDS (intensity of pain or discomfort) 10-0 or Small, Medium, or Large.

Then tap, substituting in the gaps as you filled in above.

Setup:
"Even though I have this _____, I accept myself anyway".

Reminder:
"This _____."

If you struggle to say "I accept myself anyway", simply replace it with "I just want to feel better".

As an example, Jan feels an intensity of itchiness of about a 3 out of 10. He can say something like this.

Setup:
"Even though I have this itch on the inside of my right wrist, I accept myself anyway."

If he struggles to say "I accept myself anyway", he sees that replacing it with "I just want to feel better" feels more comfortable for him, so he does.

Reminder:
"This feeling about this itch on the inside of my right wrist."

Jan does this twice, then re-assesses what level of itchiness he has on the inside of his right wrist. He may be surprised to find it has gone down to zero, but that he now has an itchiness of scale 2 on his right thumb.

This is a good sign, as it kind of means that the energy disruption is finding its way out of his body. So Jan changes his statement accordingly.

Jan now taps for "this itchiness on my right thumb". He repeats the tapping with the new statement, and after a few times, the itchiness is gone.

Now, you tap the procedure once, repeat again, then...

Evaluate your SUDS 10-0 or Small, Medium, or Large.

Evaluate how the pain/discomfort/challenge has changed. Where is it now? Has it changed in quality? Has it changed in severity in the same place, or is it different in some other way?

Keep repeating the tapping like Jan did until you reach a SUDS of 2 or less or Small or less, or preferably zero. If you cannot get to a 2 or less, just get down to the lowest number that you can on this occasion.

Physical issues do have a habit of returning when we only tap on the physical symptoms. However, it is easy to keep tapping 5-10 minutes a few times a day, and you may find that the pain,/ discomfort, or challenge eventually disappears.

Sometimes this disappears in 5 minutes never to return, and sometimes regular tapping becomes a simple pain management routine.

Sometimes, the pain is a kind of marker or imprint of the trauma suffered by the mind-body and does not shift until this trauma is released. This is when it is recommended to work with an experienced practitioner to release the trauma, if it is too much.

But not every situation is straightforward. Let me remind you of my pain story. I used to get terrible neck pain. I was almost always on pain medication and also visited an osteopath, a physiotherapist, and a massage therapist way more than my health plan or budget allowed for. Then I discovered EFT. The first thing I ever tapped for was this neck pain. When it reduced to something like a 2 or 1 out of 10, I kept tapping excitedly till it totally went. I was ecstatic. I was like a kid with a new toy. The pain reappeared every few hours at the beginning, and I promptly tapped it all the way back to zero again.

I kept tapping like this for 3 months. Yes, 3 months of tapping every few hours. Then one day, I noticed that I woke up without any of the pain. Then a few months later, I realized that I dad not tapped for that pain for weeks, because it was not there anymore.

Sometimes we need **persistence**.

I am so glad that I did persist.

Despite actual physical injuries in that area requiring a chiropractic or other manipulation about once a year or so, I am free of pain, unless I am very stressed by having to do boring admin or editing or anything that feels like a pain in the neck. But that is a rare occurrence, I am delighted to report!

Remember, persistence pays great dividends. You can do this. And you can enjoy the benefits.

CHAPTER 14 - MORE SPECIFICITY

Let us look more deeply into the emotional parts of this pain. What irritates you? What weighs you down? What emotional thing do you find hard to digest? Do you carry the world on your shoulders? Who just can't get off your back? What or/who do you find a pain in the neck? Who stabbed you in the back? Who or what is a pain in the backside?

Time and time again, I find that there is an emotional component to physical pain. It may be big or it may be small, but releasing it is the easiest part for most people.

Muscles, joints, organs, and even your cells are now thought by some to have a memory. Your muscles can even be locked into an event that your conscious mind has long forgotten.

Your body makes chemicals in response to stresses such as fear or feeling angry. If you produce more than your body can handle, it makes sense that it can increase pain.

So, ask yourself: "What irritates me?" Common emotional pain components are listed below.

An event that preceded or accompanied the pain, such as a physical accident or an emotional event.
Rejection
Fear
Unexpressed anger
Guilt

Shame

Frustration

For each of these emotions, list 5 separate actual event that typify these emotions. For example, Mary's rejection events are:

The time when Laura and Errol ambushed her outside school and stole her phone.
The time when Mary's ex John said he wanted to finish their relationship.
The last time that Mary's mother was dismissive in a phone conversation.
Last Tuesday in the restaurant when the waiter put Mary at the worst table.
Two years ago in January when Mary got sacked from her job.

Now list yours. But we are not listing them just for insights. We are listing them so that we can release them. EFT is a great way to remove negative emotions.

To give you examples of how to proceed, let us make EFT Statements for Mary's rejection. For simplicity, I will illustrate with the last example. This is two years ago in January when Mary got sacked from her job.

Setup:
"Even though I got the sack from work two years ago in January, I accept myself anyway"

Reminder:
"Got the sack from work two years ago in January"

Mary taps on this specific incident until it has no intensity for her. It may take one minute, one hour, or one month. It does not matter how long. Persistence and perseverance pay great dividends. When this event has no intensity for Mary, she moves onto the next one, and so on.

There are other ways to get specific. And of course, when there is a pain that stubbornly reappears, Mary can use the following tapping until the pain subsides.

To use these statements for yourself, simply substitute for the body part. For example, if the pain is on the right side of your neck, where it says "[body part where the pain is]", substitute "right side of my neck".

Setup:
"Even though I have this pain in my [body part where the pain is], I accept myself anyway"
(Or "... I just want to feel better")

Reminder:
"This pain in my [body part where the pain is]"

So if Mary's pain is being felt in her neck on the right, her statements would become as follows.

Setup:
"Even though I have this pain in my neck on the right, I accept myself anyway"

Reminder:
"This pain in my neck on the right"

As well as working on specific events and being specific on where the pain is, Mary can use a positive EFT tapping each morning and night, just before waking and just before going to sleep, for four weeks. She taps on all the points the following.

Setup and Reminder:
"I choose to release all the emotional components of this pain and everything they remind me of. I choose to do this until I am free from these emotions. I allow healing to my mind and body."

Now make up your own EFT protocol.

Enjoy the release...

Advanced EFTers can also tap for foods, rehabilitation exercise, etc. For example, if you have a slight allergy-like reaction to milk or gluten, well, they can be hard to avoid. So we can be specific and hold a container with some milk or wheat in it and tap as follows:

Setup:
"Even though I have this reaction to [substance], I accept myself anyway"

Reminder:
"This reaction to [substance]"

This can help the tapper with their allergy-like reactions and can help them to eat foods that are kinder to their pain levels.

If tapping for substances, choose one or two at a time and tap for them daily for a week. The next week, choose another one or two and do the same.

To illustrate the mind-body connection, let me tel you about Pat, with gratitude to Pat for sharing her story.

Pat contacted me for EFT following a stroke. I was due to give an advanced EFT workshop involving EFT for pain and mobility, so I invited her as a volunteer. Pat was 85 at the time of that first session. She subsequently had four more sessions with me. In total, the sessions were over a two month period.

Pat came in totally dependent on her walking stick. Her issue started upon the death of her sister, when Pat got vertigo. A year later, she had a stroke, after which she could hardly walk. Pat was close to her sister, whom she described as the left brain of the two, Pat being the right brain sister. Pat was the creative one. Her sister gave her advice and guidance about the logical things in life.

Because of this, we decided to challenge Pat's left and right coordination. It had been less than six months since the stroke. Peter, a student in my class who is a rehabilitation and pain expert, said that this meant there was still a good chance of developing neural connections to aid recovery. In the tapping, we bilaterally (both sides) tapped the EFT shortcut sequence ending it short at the Collarbone, as Pat said she did not like tapping on the Under Arm point.

Then we did the 9-Gamut, and we finished with the same sequence.

If you want to learn the 9-Gamut as part of the EFT Tapping, you can find it on my YouTube channel here: https://youtu.be/0D1bJenWIm4?si=Ca601Nyq3y5OhJNi or just go to the EFT Course playlist at https://www.youtube.com/@EFT-Tapping-Course-and-Videos and watch "EFT Course Lesson 2 – Setup and Reminder".

Anyway, you can do this without the 9-Gamut, as most EFT practitioners completely leave it out and still get great results. All the scientific research into EFT is without the 9-gamut.

Pat tapped on herself following our lead, and we tapped on the Gamut point of the left hand in one round, then on the Gamut point of the right hand in the next, alternating each time. At first it was a challenge for Pat to tap in this alternate way. By the end of the session, she was doing it with ease. We tapped only relatively little in this two-hour session with great progress.

We started working straight away on sister grief issues. We did not ask for her level of intensity on this occasion, as it seemed inappropriate at this stage. Pat first had anger and resentment for her sister. The first issue that came up for the grief surprised me, but we worked with it anyway. Her sister, being the logical thinker, had suggested sending Pat's son to boarding school which was "disastrous". So we tapped, with the Setup statements beginning something like as follows.

Even though she sent him to boarding school...

Even though I have this resentment towards my sister...

Even though I can't forgive her...

Even though I have lost my left brain...

Interestingly enough, this corresponded to the physical issue of Pat's stroke. Then we continued tapping something like...

Even though I have lost my sister, I choose to stand up on my own now.

We then moved onto the level of intensity scale. We wanted to rate how challenging walking without a stick was to Pat. Pat decided on a scale where 10 was the easiest and 0 the worst.

Whereas we usually have 10 as the hardest and 0 as the easiest, the opposite was Pat's choice, so we stuck to it.

Pat walked about 3 yards or just under 3 metres, turned, and walked back. She rated this a 3.5 out of 10, with 10 being the easiest, and found it hard to keep her balance. We tapped.

Even though it's hard to keep my balance...

Even though I feel I'm going to fall...

After each tapping, Pat would get up and walk the same walk again. The numbers for ease of walking this distance went up to 4.5 then to 5. Pat felt wobbly. And Peter noticed that her feet turned inwards when she stood or walked. In his experience, this indicated that the piriformis muscles (part of the connection between hip and leg) were weak. Pat also found the turning around hard to do and less than a 5. Peter found this to be connected to the left shoulder being too high and the left leg seeming too long. We tapped some more.

Even though my feet turn in...

Even though my left shoulder is too high...

Even though my left leg is too long...

Afterwards, the turn was a 5 too. I gave the feet and shoulder statements to Pat for homework. I got so excited, I forgot to write the 0-10 intensity level at the end of this session! Pat walked out without the use of the stick.

Pat continued to improve. She went through a bit of a hiccup when a bus she was on suddenly braked and she consequently fell, but our last session took care of that.

And the next chapter has very easy instructions with regards to physical rehabilitation.

CHAPTER 16 – REHABILITATION TAPPING

With rehabilitation after some kind of injury or trauma, you may have seen a physiotherapist or other physical therapist who gave you rehabilitation exercises to do. Now, we all know that they may be boring, tedious, and even possibly painful. But doing them works. So, before you do your physio exercise, you can tap as follows, using whichever description works for you, for example, "boring" or "painful" or "tedious". Choose one, or use whatever word comes to you.

Setup:
"Even though I don't feel like doing this boring/painful/tedious exercise, I just want to feel better."

Reminder:
"This boring/painful/tedious exercise"

Keep tapping until you start doing the exercise. If you feel deflated again, just repeat the tapping. You can be pleasantly surprised how motivating this can be!

Of course, not all pain is due to injuries or damage. Some of us have a regular pain that comes and goes at certain times, like period pain. Or like neck and shoulder stiffness for someone who has just spent a great deal of time working at their computer. Or pain from a workout where you just took things a bit too far.

What follows in the next chapter is another, simpler, case study that you may find helpful.

CHAPTER 16 – MOIRA

"Moira" (not her real name) remembers a time when she was rushed to hospital with suspected appendix trouble. She was terrified and literally doubled up in pain whilst waiting to be seen. After all the necessary tests were done, it was decided that she was simply having a very painful period. It was her worst ever.

It is not uncommon for women to have period pain. A pain relief tablet can be such a boon at that time. However, women are looking for natural alternatives. And EFT is just such a solution.

Moira does EFT occasionally when she gets period pain. However, since becoming a regular tapper on anything that comes up for healing, she found that her periods have become much less painful. Some are slightly uncomfortable, and others go without incident. So how does this work and what do you need to do?

Well, it is known that when we are tense, our muscles get more tense. And the more tense our muscles, the more likely it is that we feel pain. When we relax, our muscles relax. And relaxed muscles mean minimal or no pain.

EFT is a great way of letting go of tension. The simplest thing to tap for whenever period pain presents itself is as follows.

Setup:
"Even though I have this period pain, I accept myself anyway"

(Or "Even though I have this period pain, I just want to feel better")

Reminder:
"This period pain"

Simply tap until the pain goes away completely or recedes to a minimum.

Moira tapped for her period pain when she got it. She did not tap for the period pain itself when she was not experiencing it. Remember that tapping for pain needs to be when you are feeling the pain. The same principle applies for any pain, not just period pain.

I hope this example helps.

The next chapter contains a very important concept. I highly recommend that you read and digest it.

CHAPTER 17 – AN IMPORTANT EFT CONCEPT - CHASING THE PAIN

Chasing the pain is literally to tap and tap as you feel the pain "move itself" out of your body. You do this until it is gone or gets as low as you can get it.

Here are the main steps:

Where do you feel it in your body? If you get a physical pain, tap as suggested in the previous chapters.

If you do not feel a physical but an emotional pain and do not get body sensations for emotional events, do not worry. The same applies if you feel the pain in one area only and it stays exactly there as you tap until it is gone or much reduced. **If pain always stays in the same place and does not shift to other places in your body**, you can totally skip this whole module and **be a proficient EFTer all the same.**

This technique can be used for physical or emotional pain that manifests somewhere in your body, such as in your tummy, your throat, your head, etc. If you do feel an emotional or physical pain that moves to a new area as you tap for it, you can chase it till it finally leaves your body.

Imagine the pain is like a cloud of "energy". See it in your **mind's eye** becoming lighter and looser. Allow it to find its way out of your body. Become a curious observer. **Ask** yourself, with a **light sense of curiosity**, where the pain will go on its way out of your body. Notice the next body part it goes to. **Comgratulate** yourself for moving this pain. You are moving it and allowing it to travel to its way out. That is the visualisation or **concept you can have in your mind as you tap.**

Observe it leaving, become an observer. Let it go, safely and calmly, and that is perfectly OK.

As always, keep a measure of the intensity of the pain in that particular area. And re-assess after each round of tapping.

When the pain moves to a different area, it may be at a lower or higher intensity. If higher, do not worry. This is normal. Carry on tapping. If the pain then moves again, keep tapping. Between each tapping round, measure the intensity of pain again. Carry on like this until the pain no longer moves and is at the lowest intensity you can get.

There is no need to get worked up about where to call the location of the pain. You can simply refer to it as "just there". **As long as you know in your mind where "just there" is, that is perfectly OK.**

Here are some more varied wordings for you to use. Choose the ones that resonate best with you. After all, it is all about you feeling good as a result!

Setup:

"Even though I have this pain just there, I accept myself anyway" (Or you can say "Even though I have this pain just there, I just want to feel better")

Reminder:

"This pain just there"

... Or... (substitute for the words in between the []...

Setup: "Even though I have this [feeling] in my [body part], I accept myself anyway"...

Reminder: "This [feeling] in my [body part]"

Chase the pain as it moves around the body. This could be a physical OR emotional pain, for example, a pain in the lower back on the right or a fear in the stomach.

Remember, **if** you end up with a headache, chase the pain out of your head too. You can say as follows...

Setup:

"Even though I have this headache, I just want to let it go"

Reminder:

"This headache"

Repeat till gone. Once you get used to chasing the pain, you can find it very useful.

CHAPTER 18 - COMPLEX PAIN EXAMPLE

The following EFT Tapping procedure is from my own personal experience quite a while back, when I was still building my client base. Note my negative language at the beginning. In fact, the whole experience that I tapped as I wrote about it was released, and I successfully repeating the same client building marketing exercise later on. In other words, both the physical and emotional pain were released.

This procedure illustrates my thinking as I was doing the EFT Tapping for a pain in my right shoulder. My right shoulder had been through a physical mishap many years before in a gym accident. However, I only felt pain there when overloaded with emotional stress.

In this case, the emotional stress was about a marketing campaign in my work. Your pain may be related to a personal issue, a work issue, or anything. I included this case in this book to give you an ideas for your tapping, if needed.

"Last night, my spouse said that I kept talking over and over again about how distressed I was. Of course, due to client confidentiality, I could not reveal anything. Today, I have many tasks ahead of me, admin and customer service, and I just have totally lost the confidence to do them. And my right shoulder keeps migrating towards my ear

due to the sheer stress of it all, and that creates unbelievable pain. So, I am letting go of most of this morning's tasks and spending quality time tapping here. I cannot move forward in this state. I need to let it go. I want to let it go.

"Pain 9 out of 10, despite having taken an anti-inflammatory (something I very rarely resort to but had to use often during this marketing ordeal) and used Epsom salts and a massage on that area. So I tap...

"Setup:
'Even though I am carrying [that particularly sad and despairing] pain in my right shoulder, it is the marketing campaign's pain, I just want to let it go. I am not responsible for the marketing campaign's pain. I can make the choice and decision to accept it is what it is. I accept without judgment.'

"I tapped this Setup 3-4 times. Pain down to 6.5 out of 10. Before I got to the Reminder, I could see an image of myself in my mind. It was during a particularly sad and despairing part of this campaign, looking sad and helpless, my face devoid of any joy, my body slumped and tense at the same time. I look all black. My hair is black, my clothes are black, my skin is black (not brown or any shade of normal human skin color but actually pitch black), my eyes are totally black all over. So I tap for the woman in the picture. I tap for me in that situation, in total black despair and depression...

"Setup:
'Even though I am carrying [that marketing campaign]'s pain in my right shoulder, it is the campaign pain, I just want to let it go. I am not responsible for this pain., I can make the choice and decision to accept the situation. I accept without judgment. Even though it is giving me this total black despair and deep depths of depression, I want to get out of this state. I want to free this woman (myself in that picture) from her pain. She wants to be free from her pain. I love her very much'

"I did this setup once and saw myself still totally black, now curled up in the fetal position, scared and just wanting help asap. I look at her

(the me in that picture) and tap on her behalf...

"Setup:
'Your blackness, Your curled-up-ness. I love you anyway'.

"Reminder:
'Your blackness, Your curled-up-ness. I love you anyway' ... tapping and crying... Reminder only, over and over again, as many rounds as I want, also adding the 9-Gamut, as it really helps me: "Your blackness, Your curled-up-ness. I love you anyway"

"Pain down to 3 out of 10. I am back to being in the colors I was wearing at that session, my hair is back to blonde, my face and skin and eyes are back to their color at that session. I am no longer curled up. I am still slumped. Now tapping for both me and her (the me in that particular session)... Reminder only, over and over again, as many rounds as I want: 'My pain in my shoulder just there, Your slump-ness, your fear, your despair. I love you anyway'.

"She is now fine. I have this pain in my shoulder now down to 2, and I feel it is because of anger. I am angry with myself for having invested in this particular marketing program instead of another, which in retrospect would have been a lot easier on me, although with this one, I was guaranteed financial success and the other one carried no guarantees. I should have taken that risk.

"Setup and reminder: 'This anger in my shoulder just there, I just want to let it go.'

"Pain down to a 1 out of 10. Stretching... Stretching some more... Doing shoulder mobilization exercises... Pain down to 0. Old injury around T3 in my back feels like a 0.5, so the pain has moved there but is minimal. I have the confidence to carry on with my next task now, which is mega-urgent and one that pleases me. I will tap again later when I have the time. For now, I can function and carry on with my work for the day. I will be happy and satisfied."

This whole tapping took just over an hour, just to give you an idea of what to expect for slightly complex pain.

I hope this story inspired you to do your own detective work for complex pain.

And as you can see, I did not stick to the more classical form of doing EFT but let it lead me using imagery and healing that image of myself in the suffering situation. EFT is very flexible. If you want to add wording that has helped you with pain in the past or techniques that have helped you from elsewhere, by all means you can use them whilst tapping.

Most of all, remember the two main important parts to making EFT work best for you:
1.   Be as specific as you can;
2.   Be persistent. Persistence helps. Even if you only do the simplest form of EFT over and over again, you can get results.

And it is all about results.

CHAPTER 19 – "ENERGY TOXINS" EFT TAPPING KRYPTONITE

EFT Tapping works for the vast majority of people. Someone who has had remarkable results with EFT Tapping can recommend it to a friend, and the friend would think that's crazy, because it did nothing for them. Every now and then, on the very rare occasion (maybe 0.5 % of clients), I get a client whose numbers go down painfully slowly, and whose results do not hold from one session to the next. So, what is happening?!

Although it usually means that we did not get specific enough in our statements, there is a rare few people who have what is termed an "energy toxin". In my client experience, this usually boils down to one of two reasons:

1.   The person is, despite their efforts, undernourished with regards to foods that help their nervous system work well enough for EFT Tapping to work.
2.   The person, despite having no symptoms, has a kind of allergy-like reaction to a certain foodstuff.

In both of these cases that are in my client experience, the effect is sub-clinical. That means the problem is at such a small level that it is not detectable by the average medical test. I have sent clients who were open to investigating their diets to nutritionists, kinesiologists, or bioresonance practitioners, who helped them identify the issue. Of those clients who chose to work with the practitioner and follow their advice, 100% were able to get good results afterwards with EFT Tapping.

With physical pain, sometimes the pain keeps returning, even though every time you tap for it it goes down significantly in intensity.

This does not indicate an energy toxin.

Remember that when I started my EFT Tapping journey, I tapped several times a day for a particular physical pain. Every time, it would reduce from a high intensity to a zero. The pain would be back to the high intensity in about 3-4 hours. After 3 months of this, the results held for longer than a few hours. Within a few more weeks, the results held for good, despite actual damage in that region of my body. I **did not** have an energy toxin.

With an energy toxin, you would only go down by a 0.5-1 points out of 10 in intensity, or perhaps one day this happens but the next day it does not budge. Or maybe you do not even get a reduction of 0.5 in intensity, no matter how much you tap.

If you suspect that you have an energy toxin, maybe you can contact a good nutritionist, ideally a functional nutritionist. Or contact a systemic kinesiologist or bioresonance practitioner.

Please note that energy toxins are very rare. I hope this helps.

CHAPTER 20 - THANK YOU AND TILL WE MEET AGAIN...

Thank you for buying this book, and I hope you have enjoyed using it as much as I have enjoyed making it!

To summarize, this is how we use EFT to let go of pain:

We get specific on the pain

If we are in pain, we tap for the pain we are experiencing right now.

We tap for possible root causes and stresses.

We can simply use the same basic EFT formula over and over again.

We may get rid of our pain in one tapping, or it may be a case of pain management. Either way, it is more desired these days than taking a pain-relief pill.

We can use EFT to help motivate us to take further action, such as physiotherapy exercises.

Persistence works.

Lastly, thanks again for getting this book. I hope you have enjoyed your journey to a more comfortable, happier you.

Wishing you health and happiness always...